WEIGHT LOSS AND DIET
WEIGHT LOSS AND KEEPING IT OFF SUCCESSFULLY

AUTHOR

FRANCINE BROWN

Copyright 2020 © Francine Brown

Legal & Disclaimer

The information contained in this book and its contents is not designed to replace or take the place of any form of medical or professional advice; and is not meant to replace the need for independent medical, financial, legal or other professional advice or services, as may be required. The content and information in this book has been provided for educational and entertainment purposes only.

The content and information contained in this book has been compiled from sources deemed reliable, and it is accurate to the best of the Author's knowledge, information and belief. However, the Author cannot guarantee its accuracy and validity and cannot be held liable for any errors and/or omissions. Further, changes are periodically made to this book as and when needed. Where appropriate and/or necessary, you must consult a professional (including but not limited to your doctor, attorney, financial advisor or such other professional advisor) before using any of the suggested remedies, techniques, or information in this book.

Upon using the contents and information contained in this book, you agree to hold harmless the Author from and against any damages, costs, and expenses, including any legal fees potentially resulting from the application of any of the information provided by this book. This disclaimer applies to any loss, damages or injury caused by the use and application, whether directly or indirectly, of any advice or information presented, whether for breach of contract, tort, negligence, personal injury, criminal intent, or under any other cause of action. You agree to accept all risks of using the information presented inside this book.

You agree that by continuing to read this book, where appropriate and/or necessary, you shall consult a professional (including but not limited to your doctor, attorney, or financial advisor or such other advisor as needed) before using any of the suggested remedies, techniques, or information in this book.

Table of Contents

INTRODUCTION

Losing weight is never an easy process, but a more infuriating process is to come to terms with why you want to lose weight. Several factors, such as body image issues, health issues, overweight problems, bullying, or peer pressure, contribute to losing weight. First off, you must understand that you're perfect just the way you are, and if you want to do this, then do it for yourself only.

There are many ways on the internet, magazines, and even books on how to reduce weight. I understand the frustration you must feel when nothing seems to work for you. Don't worry, I know this is a complicated process, but this book is here to guide you through it.

Your weight loss problems end here. No more feeling ashamed or sorry for yourself and hiding on the sidelines. Get ready to meet a healthy and confident you.

CHAPTER 1

You are Not Alone

Everyone struggles with the idea of looking better. And it's okay! You don't necessarily have to feel 'good about yourself' all the time. It is okay to have doubts, and it's okay to want to be better- that's the only way you improve.

Losing weight can be a grueling process. You have to make unimaginable changes to your diet and throttle most of your cravings. 5 in 10 people today are trying to lose weight. Furthermore, 60% of the overweight population is intent on shedding their extra pounds. So, guess what? You're not the only one.

I want you to lose your weight without losing your senses, which is why this comprehensive book will let you in on some of the unknown secrets of weight loss. I will take you to step by step through various stages of this journey and help you form a singular plan as per the needs of your body. Let's begin!

CHAPTER 2

Body Types and Personalized Weight Loss

Even after you've been exercising and eating well, you might not get the results you want. This is because people rely on universal weight loss plans without recognizing how their body is made.

The idea of various body types comes from 40s doctor- William Herbert Sheldon. The type of body you have can give you an insight into your metabolism and hormones. This will help you analyze the amount of protein, carbs, and other nutrients you need.

Your body type also goes on to affect your mood. This knowledge can be successfully incorporated in your routine to fasten the process of weight loss.

How to Identify Your Body Type

There are three different body types. Your daily exercise and metabolic changes determine these. For women, even menopause goes on to affect their body type. Many people feel that external factors have significantly affected their bodies. For them, I recommend looking back into teen and childhood years.

Once you've done this, consider the list below-

1)   **Endomorph-** Endomorphs have more body fat. Women in this category are usually curvaceous, while men are rather stocky. If you are an endomorph, your weight will be concentrated in your things, hips, and belly. This body type needs to watch the carbohydrate intake.

2)   **Ectomorph-** Long, thin, and bony. Ectomorphs have a small bone structure. Further, if you are an ectomorph, your shoulders will be narrower as compared to your hips. This body

type has trouble gaining weight and can handle more carbohydrates.

3)   Mesomorph- If you are a mesomorph, you will have a medium frame with an hourglass figure. Also, your muscles will be considerably prominent.

Here's a quiz to help you assess your body type.

Other than the three main body types mentioned above, there are also certain hybrids. For example-

Ecto-Mesomorph- Lean and Muscular

Meso-Endomorphs- Strong, undefined muscles

Ecto- Endomorphs- Skinny fat as a result of inadequate exercise

WEIGHT-LOSS FOR DIFFERENT BODY TYPES

Determining your somatotype and where it falls helps determine nutrient intake. What more, it keeps you safe from any such diet plans which might backfire. For instance, Ectomorphs do well with a high carbohydrate plan and Endomorphs with a protein-rich diet.

Working with your body type is crucial because it helps you maximize your limitations. Moreover, it ensures that you do not get too frustrated too soon. Let's deal with different body types one by one.

Endomorph

Weight-loss plans for endomorphs should focus mainly on reducing fat and improving cardio-respiratory efficiency. It is also recommended to incorporate resistance training and focus on strengthening the muscles.

Diet and Weight Loss

The best diet plan for endomorphs comes from a moderate distribution of macronutrients. Also, all the carbohydrates should come from vegetables in contrast to high-fiber starch like quinoa. Keep a distance from cookies, crackers, cereal, and bread.

A Paleo-diet best suits an endomorph. This meal plan includes healthy fats like avocado, olive oil, as well as vegetables, and protein. Try to get a nutrition distribution with 30% carbs, 35% fat, and 35% protein.

Additionally, jump-start your day with a protein-rich breakfast to boost metabolism. This also ensures that your insulin levels stay controlled. Your diet should contain as much as 2.2 grams of protein per kilogram of body weight. This supports existing muscle tissue at the time of calorie restriction.

After you have ensured that the daily protein requirement has been met, try to blend carbs and fats. A 'keto' diet might help some people to burn more fat throughout the day. However, this isn't recommended for people who experience symptoms of nausea.

The most crucial step is determining your calorie intake throughout the day. After this, you need to lower your food intake slightly and limit the calories you take.

Sample Diet for Endomorphs

Stick to dividing your diet between carbohydrates, protein, and fat in the ratio 20:40:40. Try to take grains with dinner or lunch-depending on your workout.

- **Breakfast-** Spinach and Eggs
- **Snack:** Multigrain protein bar
- **Lunch-** Roasted lamb lettuce wraps
- **Snack-** Hummus and vegetables
- **Dinner-** Quinoa and zucchini noodles with chicken

Endomorphs are more inclined to relax and take things easy. But they must remember to incorporate motion in their everyday activities. Cardio training is exceptionally essential for endomorphs to burn calories. Furthermore, this ensures that they can maintain a calorie deficit.

Try and incorporate HIIT or high-intensity interval training two or three times a week. Do this for 20-30 minutes of every workout. Also, incorporate 60 and 30 minutes of steady-state cardio twice or thrice a week.

Weight Training

It is essential to build and maintain lean muscle mass while getting rid of body fat. You also need to rev up your metabolism, which should be the main focus of your weight-training sessions. Developing your muscle tissues will help to increase metabolic rate while resting while burning more fat.

Focus on the larger muscle groups like the back or legs. Include high repetitions throughout the workout. Also include circuit training and compound exercises with less time gap between various sets.

Losing fat with only your diet is a little difficult for endomorphs. Exercise is crucial to boost your metabolism, which needs both cardio and weight training.

Building muscles is not difficult for this body type. However, the unneeded body fat ant and slow metabolism make it a bit difficult for endomorphs to stay lean. Try to incorporate different activities daily to prevent boredom.

Ectomorph

Ectomorphs face challenges that are entirely opposite to those faced by endomorphs. This body type has a highly active metabolism with bony bone structures. This makes it hard for them to gain weight and keep it on. This is why cardio-respiratory plans are meant to reduce the overall utilization of energy.

Diet and Weight Loss

Ectomorphs are blessed with a fast metabolism. This makes it easy for them to stay lean and eat anything they want without worrying about getting fat. Although with age, metabolism tends to slow down due to muscle mass. Consequently, they end up gaining some unwanted mass.

The perfect diet for an ectomorph is one that has high calories and carbohydrates. The distribution of calories should be in the ratio 50:25:25 for carbs, fat, and protein, respectively. Some tips every ectomorph should follow:

- Eat every second or fourth hour.

- Consume at least 500 calories if you want to gain muscle or weight.

- Pick warm food over cold as it is better for digestion.

- The best carbs are starchy ones—potatoes, sweet potatoes, quinoa, brown rice, and oats.

- The best fruits are peaches, avocado, papaya, pineapple, mangoes, and bananas.

- Best vegetables include carrots, beets, Brussel sprouts, cauliflower, and broccoli.

The most important thing is to remember and take all the possible nutrients. Also, right before your workout, try to take a carbohydrate, which is easy to digest. Don't forget to take an adequate amount of water before and after the workout.

The best post-workout snack should have a 1:3 ratio of proteins to carbs. This is important to build and repair muscle fiber while replenishing glycogen levels.

Ectomorphs have to eat moderate amounts of protein, high amounts of carbohydrate, and lesser fat—the ideal split 50-25-25, as mentioned above.

- **Breakfast-** Nuts and fruits with oatmeal

- **Snack 1-** Protein Shake

- **Lunch-** Vegetable salad with vinaigrette, chicken, and chopped veggies

- **Snack 2-** Almonds and Apples

- **Dinner-** Quinoa with broccoli and grilled shrimp

Cardio

Most ectomorphs will pick cardio training overweight lifting. This is because the body type does well with endurance-related activities. If you want to initiate muscle growth, it is essential to do minimal cardio. Only do that much as is needed for the general health of your body.

I recommend that you indulge in cardio three times a week for no longer than 30 minutes. Maximal strength training and hypertrophy are always better than cardio. Firstly, these are mostly anaerobic, and secondly, they do not instigate fast calorie burn up when resting.

Ectomorphs must have a simple weight training routine with heavyweights. The focus is primarily on weightlifting and completing three to five sets. Moreover, these sets should have eight or twelve reps for every muscle group.

With the help of balanced energy intake, lifting, and strength training, it helps ectomorphs build their body mass.

Keep in Mind

Ectomorphs find themselves at a disadvantage when trying to sculpt their bodies or build muscles. Therefore, a dedicated nutrition and training program is needed to sculpt and create curves on their small frame.

Ectomorphs can aim for anything- to get a healthy lean body or become a bodybuilder. But they have to take care to manage their metabolism through solid weight-training.

There's no other way around it. Mesomorphs have comparatively much more comfortable than the other two body types. They have efficient metabolisms, but their muscle mass also allows them to have a flexible fitness plan. The foundation work required by this group of people is minimal.

Diet and Weight Loss

Mesomorphs have a higher ratio of muscle. Owing to this, they have comparatively higher calorie requirements than their contemporaries. Other body types require proteins, fats, and carbohydrates in equal proportion. However, mesomorphs' bodies mostly require high-protein meals.

The best way advice is to divide nutrition equally among protein, vegetables, and whole grains. Also, include protein in every meal to help build and repair muscles. Protein sources that work best include- Greek yogurt, lentils, beans, fish, turkey, chicken, and eggs.

Carbohydrates are equally crucial since your body will require glucose to produce energy and synthesize glucose. It is best to mix the carbohydrates and have a variety of food like oatmeal, brown rice, quinoa, and whole grains. Other than this, include seasonal fruits and vegetables in your diet.

Mesomorphs can gain weight quickly with increased calorie intake. Similarly, it is equally comfortable to shed the extra pounds with a balanced diet and the right amount of exercise. If you are a mesomorph, also take care to include healthy fats like olive oil, coconut oil, avocado, seeds, and nuts.

Sample Diet for Mesomorph

Mesomorph body types should split calories between carbohydrates, fat, and protein in the ratio 30:30:40. This is the only way to shed body fat while maintaining a healthy weight. More or less, an even balance needs to be maintained between the three.

- **Breakfast-** Scrambled eggs and toast

- **Snack-** Fruit and protein bar

- **Lunch-** Salad with chickpeas, chopped veggies, and olive oil dressing

- **Snack-** Hummus and Veggies

- **Dinner-** Sweet potato, roasted veggies, and chicken breast

Cardio

If a mesomorph wants to attain a lean physique, they need to invest in consistent cardio. It is advised that you include thirty or forty-five minutes of cardiovascular workout and follow this routine three to five times a week.

If you carry less body fat, reduce the cardio sessions to two times a week. For best results, follow HIIT (high-intensity interval training) and cardio interval workouts. Incorporate these two or three times a week, along with slow, long-duration cardio.

Continuous aerobic exercise and slow cardio does not burn too many calories and goes easy on your body. It also decreases the risk of injury- all of which is essential to a workout.

Weight Training

Mesomorphs are strong naturally because their muscles are dense and think. They should concentrate on lifting heavy or moderate weights with limited rests. Take out five days a week to stimulate muscle development.

Moreover, it is vital to perform 8-12 reps of three exercises for every muscle group. After you complete three sets of every exercise, take a break of thirty to ninety seconds. Also, switch your training routine and include high reps with light weights.

Add in a body-weight workout along with circuit training and supersets. All these combined will help develop stamina and strength without increasing muscle mass.

KEEP IN MIND

Both men and women with a mesomorph body type can quickly build muscle. However, they have a slight tendency to gain weight and have a focus on a well-rounded workout and balanced diet to maintain a lean physique.

Mesomorphs are genetically favored when it comes to building muscles. If you aim to stay lean and slim, focus on your cardio and diet.

CHAPTER 3

How Can You Effectively Lose Weight To Maintain A Wholesome And Energetic Lifestyle?

According to the World Health Organization (WHO), about 13% of the world's population in 2016 were diagnosed with obesity. It is a type of health problem that can give rise to multiple health issues. For instance, hypertension, diabetes, cardiac distress, sleep-related issues, etc., are commonly linked to obesity.

Furthermore, it has an adverse effect on our lifestyle and personality. You can lose the ability to run, to walk extra miles, or even sit comfortably. The only solution to all of these problems is losing extra pounds of weight in a healthy manner.

Losing weight is only advised if you are obese or want to feel fit. You should do it for yourself and not for anyone else. Remember this- there is no shame in cutting down extra weight by religiously following an active weight loss plan.

In the following issue of healthy weight loss, you will find crucial tips and information to help you achieve your desired weight goal. The traditional advice which is given by all dieticians and nutritionists is to reduce food intake. However, it is not as easy as it sounds and takes a strong mindset to refuse the tempting sugary and junk food.

One vital point to remember when you're reducing your food intake to an optimum amount is not to do it quickly. Sudden changes in the food intake can take a toll on your mental health and hamper the overall results. Take baby steps and go easy on yourself.

Moreover, reduction of food intake does not mean you stop eating altogether. It means you cut down on junk and other unhealthy food and instead switch to fruits and vegetables. Dairy products that are low-fat, pulses, whole grains combined with a minimum 8-10 glasses of water are the thumb rule of a healthy and balanced diet.

Eating healthy is only step 1 of losing weight. The second step is to exercise or work out vigorously. To achieve your desired weight goal, you have to push yourself to follow a fitness regime.

Not only is exercising beneficial to your body, but it is also an effective way to melt those extra layers of fat. Try to spend a minimum of 30 minutes on physical activity to burn calories, increase stamina, and tone your muscles. These activities can range from Zumba, going to the gym, walking, jogging, or home workout sessions.

Whatever alternative you choose, it will require commitment both physically and mentally. There is no easy way out. You need to work hard and remain motivated if you want to get rid of those extra pounds.

The path to healthily losing weight is difficult, but the end result is worth it. Every minute of working out and every vegetable that you ate will contribute to your weight loss plan. I guarantee that at the end of this journey, you will be both physically and mentally fit.

Maintaining Weight Loss

It is possible to accomplish weight loss with several modalities. However, it is far more challenging to sustain this long-term weight loss. Obesity treatments usually lead to accelerated weight reduction accompanied by weight plateau and eventual regain. Studies even show that more than

Obesity management includes comprehensive professional care, along with weight-specific therapy. These are crucial to promoting lifelong eating practices and effective weight control.

WHY ARE PEOPLE OBESE?

Continued weight control is particularly challenging owing to our evolutionary, behavioral, and obesogenic climate experiences. The spike in the incidence of obesity in the last few decades became reflected through the industrialization of the food supply. This includes a rise in the manufacturing and selling of inexpensive, highly refined products that viciously accelerate the appetite.

Ultra-processed food contributes to several calories among consumers today. Some reasons why you could be obese-

- Eating fast food or processed food in large amounts.

- Consuming excessive alcohol and sugary drinks

- Less consumption of healthy, homemade meals

- Eating more than your body demands

- Comfort eating

Furthermore, a shift in the physical movement culture has rendered it increasingly difficult to remain healthy all day. Working sectors have become increasingly sedentary, while vehicular transportation is favored over walking.

HOW TO OVERCOME A WEIGHT PLATEAU

After you lose weight, your metabolism declines considerably. This causes you to burn lesser calories than you initially did at a heavier weight. Your slow metabolism decreases your weight loss. This happens even if you eat the same number of calories that made weight loss possible. Once you reach the stage where calories consumed equals calories burnt, it is known as the weight plateau.

However, there are some simple ways to dodge this phenomenon. For instance-

- **Assessing your habits again-** Examine the history of your meals and activities. Try to ensure you don't loosen the rules by doing less exercise for a long time.

- **Cutting calories-** Decrease your calories, but don't let them go below 1200 in a day. If you do this, you run the risk of binge eating or overeating.

- **Increasing the workout-**People should exercise at least 30 minutes a day throughout the week. If you want to speed up your weight loss process, consider increasing the intensity of your exercise. This will help increase muscle mass.

- **Be more active-** Work outside your gym as well. Increase the amount of physical activity in general.

Losing weight can be considerably difficult for most people. But what is more challenging is to keep it off once you've shed some pounds—many people who lose significant weight gain it back within 2 or 3 years.

Exercise and dieting are essential strategies for maintaining the ideal weight for a long time. Follow the tricks and tips given in this book to attain the body you have always wanted. Regardless of what you want- becoming slimmer, or feeling healthier- these points will take you a long way.

CHAPTER 4

Dieting For Your Health And Well Being

Before you begin this journey of weight loss, you must decide if you're doing it for yourself or not. There's no point in dieting for any other reason except for yourself and your healthy lifestyle. If you are overweight, you must know that the extra weight possesses a threat to your health.

One of the similarities between smokers and most people who are overweight is addiction. Addiction is never a good thing, as too much of anything is harmful. You`re eating habits may be a result of stress eating, addiction to specific foods, or other conditioned behavior.

It is not simple, but you must push through to maintain healthy eating habits. A lot of people keep jumping the wagon from diet to another. They do so because they are not satisfied with the lack of results.

They are desperately looking for a diet that's quick and convenient. Honestly, no good can come from such expectations. You need to be kind to yourself and forgive yourself for the downfalls if you want the diet to work.

The fact is that simply following a diet plan won't magically reduce your weight. Going hard on yourself and constantly depriving yourself of treats will only harm your progress. It is okay to have a cheat day once in a while.

Remember that starving yourself will only have a negative impact on your success. It is a common myth that dieting is a golden rule to reduce weight. That again depends on what dieting means to you.

Dieting isn't starving yourself. It is simply switching to healthy and balanced meals. This is one of the positive changes many people dealing with weight problems can incorporate in their lifestyle. Another change would be to taking the stairs instead of the lift or parking your car farther away.

These simple and minute changes go a long way in your weight loss progress. It has extra physical activity in lifestyle, and you will be burning calories without realizing it. Pay attention to your daily schedule and see how many of such changes can you accommodate.

A fun suggestion for physical activity is dancing. There are ample beginner dance classes available in several dance forms for all ages and sizes. You can choose Zumba or regular dancing classes and dance your way through losing weight.

Another perk of choosing this physical activity is that it distracts yourself from hunger pangs. The extra calories burned through this psychical activity accelerates your weight loss process. Sounds fun and exciting, doesn't it?

If you feel dancing isn't your thing, then you can try other hobbies. Joining a yoga club or a walking club are good ways to socialize and lose weight. Any activity that keeps you away from the refrigerator and burning fat is good enough.

Don't forget that dieting alone is not the solution. You must combine it with any physical activity to see visible progress.

The main drawback of dieting is that people give it up too easily. People want quick results, and the lack of it makes them frustrated. Thus, they end up giving up and feel like a failure for not accomplishing enough.

No matter which diet plan you follow, it is going to take to progress. You shouldn't be too quick to mark it off as another failure without trying hard enough. Patience is the key to a successful diet.

Don't have unrealistic expectations if you weigh yourself every day to check your progress. If you are aiming to see pounds less every time you weigh yourself, then you're setting yourself up to fail.

This can lead to negative thoughts, and you will end up binge eating tubs of Bens and Jerry's. You must avoid any depressive episodes of binge eating over things like not losing 5 pounds overnight. When it comes to dieting, only a handful of them work.

Furthermore, lifestyle changes, if practiced vigorously, will 100% work. You must note that it's you who has the hard work. Any type of dieting plan will rarely lead to the desired long term goal.

CHAPTER 5

A collection of weight loss tips to boost your progress

There are several weight loss tips given by dieticians to aid you in losing weight. These tips work if followed correctly and consistently. The most predominant and critical tip is to eat healthily.

Pay attention- eating healthy doesn't refer to how much you eat. Instead, it is what you eat. Obviously, you will have to regulate the amount of food intake, but it doesn't mean that you starve yourself. When you're on a diet, focus on the food you eat, for example, switch candies with fruits.

It is advised that you do meticulous research on healthy foods. This way, you will be able to make a nutritious diet schedule and keep a count of your calories. It will give you an idea of what you can eat and what you can't.

Plain healthy eating can be tasteless and boring to some people. To avoid this, you can look at healthy recipes in cooking books or online to "spice up" your daily meals. Omit to eat the same meal continuously throughout the week. You can do so by exploring other healthy meal options.

I know you're tired of hearing about it, but it is essentially crucial to exercise or workout. The importance of physical activity cannot be stressed enough.

The body has a simple promotional rule. The number of calories that you burn, lesser will be the calorie absorbed in your body. This is what makes it possible for anyone to lose weight.

Exercising is an imperative factor to melt extra calories in your body. Just like dieting, exercising is another step that you have to take slowly. Don't burn yourself out by overdoing it.

It may be confusing about where to start, especially if you don't already have a workout regime. One handy way to plan a workout is by reading fitness magazines and blogs. They have step by step pictorial instructions on how to do the exercise and the information about its benefits.

Another way to figure out a workout routine is not watching home workout tutorials on the internet. You can also go to your local gym and get a professional trainer to tailor a workout schedule for you. Remember to start slow and don't immediately jump on to vigorous exercises.

Healthy eating and regular exercise are the perfect alliance to reduce weight. A fun tip would be to find yourself a workout partner that will keep you motivated, and it can prove to be exciting too. Both of you can together push each other to follow the routine and be a constant source of motivation.

Another way to keep yourself from being bored while working out is to frequently change your schedule. For instance, don't do the treadmill for the entire week, instead switch it up with weight lifts or cycling. Planning different exercises throughout the week will ensure that the fat stored in each part for your body is targeted.

It is okay to build up some muscle mass and tone your body. Fun fact- muscles burn fat not only when they work but also during resting. They burn calories all they long.

It is a sensible fact that you need to increase muscle mass to lose weight. Gaining muscle mass is not a complicated or far-fetched goal. You can start by choosing resistance exercise to increase the momentum of your weight loss plan.

Tracking your progress is a healthy and positive way to keep you determined, focused, and motivated. Take before and after pictures or maintain a journal about your weight loss journey. Give yourself credit by rewarding yourself with one cheat day, buying clothes, or even a movie night if you continuously followed your schedule.

Your weight loss journey doesn't have to be a tale of pain, sacrifice, and suffering. This isn't some tortuous process you have to put yourself through. It is instead of achieving a healthy lifestyle, gaining self-confidence, and freedom of doing things that you love.

Sure, this journey is filled with small or big obstacles and may require compromise here then. This doesn't mean that you have to beat yourself up every time you receive the expected results. As someone once said, "no pain, no gain."

So, pick yourself up and accommodate yourself to these few adjustments and discomforts. It might be overwhelming now, but remember your end goal. You can push through these discomforts and achieve your ultimate goal of a healthy lifestyle.

QUICK TIPS THAT WILL COME IN HANDY

Below, I have talked of six practices that will go on to help you beyond your dieting phase. Adhere to the following tips in order to avoid gaining your lost weight back.

1) Stay Hydrated

Drinking 3-4 liters of water in a day is helpful in a lot of ways. Firstly, it prevents you from feeling hungry when your body is dehydrated. Secondly, it keeps your cell active and turgid, further boosting your metabolism. Lastly, it also helps to flush down toxins like wastes and harmful oxygen species.

2) Avoid Sugar

The second crucial step is avoiding sugary food and drinks. Although it is advised to reward yourself with a treat occasionally, do not make this a habit. Celebrate your achievements by challenging yourself to do something even better.

3) Avoid Processed Food

Processed food includes microwave dinners, fast food, sugary cereals, etc. These contain unhealthy fats and sugars which accelerate weight grain. opt for healthier food instead such as- yogurt, frozen fruit, and oats.

4) Consume Veggies and Greens

Vegetables contain minerals, vitamins, fiber, antioxidants, and other phytonutrients. Not only do these rejuvenate and heal the body, but they also boost immunity and metabolism. Other benefits include the prevention of fat accumulation and reduction of blood sugar.

5) Consume Protein

Take in lean protein through tofu, mushroom, fish, turkey, soybean, chicken breast, etc. The body finds these harder to digest, thus creating a calorie deficit. It also helps you look more toned and build muscle mass

6)   Check the Ingredients

A lot of times, we end up consuming invisible calories through dressings, dips, and sauces. Other than hindering our weight loss, these also trigger the appetite to an unhealthy extent. Therefore, check all the ingredients and components of any food you buy from outside.

CHAPTER 6

Everything You Need To Know About Weight-Loss Surgery And If It's Worth It

If you aren't already aware, you can even opt for weight-loss surgery. People aiming to lose over eighty pounds, or more are eligible for weight-loss surgeries.

You might be stunned to know that you might be eligible for weight-loss surgery. However, you may also be mind-boggled about it or not it is worth it. Well, if you're wondering if you should go ahead with the surgery, here is something you should know.

The answer to if or not Weight-loss surgery is ideal for you depends on person to person. Although this doesn't exactly answer your question, deep down, only you can know the answer. Several individuals that have successfully undergone surgery suggested that it was worth it.

However, Some of them didn't encounter any benefits in the long run. In a nutshell, you may need to look into a myriad of factors before going through with the surgery. One such extremely crucial factor that goes without saying is the budget.

It comes as no surprise that weight loss surgeries are heftily priced. Thus, there is no point in putting yourself under a financial strain to get the surgery done. The cost of the surgery entirely depends on the amount of weight that you want to shred through the surgery. Moreover, most surgeons only offer surgery to those who are 80 pounds overweight. That being said, if you think you can lose weight without needing the surgery, you have your answer. If you are ready to consistently workout and eat healthily, then you are good to go.

The second and other extremely critical factor includes your health as a whole. Determining whether you should go ahead with weight loss surgery means analyzing if you are healthy enough to undergo it. Individuals with a health history should avoid surgery or consult their doctor. On the other hand, individuals who are extremely obese may need to consider otherwise.

Experts suggest that individuals who weigh extensively more than their necessary weight may even risk themselves to death. Thus, if you are severely obese, you must put your health before the costs. After all, no price tag is worth putting your health into risk.

Thirdly, motivation is an underlying factor in weight loss surgery. While the surgery may help you lose weight, you may need to consider several other factors after it. You may need to consistently workout even after the surgery.

Thus, if that's something you're willing to do, you can very well handle the surgery. Furthermore, you may need to limit yourself to junk food after a lowered tummy pouch. If not, it will only take time for you to get back to your earlier shape.

Weight loss is entirely about your determination and willpower to choose yourself over the junk. Junk food may, without a doubt, tempt you. Nonetheless, it is you who can stop yourself from going back to your unhealthy habits.

Research suggests that Bariatric surgery can help patients lose over 30 to 50% of their additional weight in the initial six months. They can further cut down 77% of their excess weight after about 12 months of the surgery. How effective is bariatric surgery? | University of Iowa Hospitals & Clinics

These sum up the very few but indispensable factors that you should consider before undergoing weight-loss surgery. While I may not be a health professional, note that weight-loss surgery entirely depends on you. I am in no way endorsing you to undergo any surgery.

I've only mentioned this to help you understand every possible option. You should consult your doctor beforehand, along with doing meticulous research.

CHAPTER 7

Using The Internet To Develop An Effective Weight-Loss Plan

Thanks to the Internet, today, we can find anything and everything we want. You can use this to your benefit for a smooth weight-loss journey. From joining weight-loss programs, doing challenges, and much more, the internet has a lot to offer.

Nutrisystem and Weight Watchers are two such explicitly famous platforms for joining weight loss programs. Nonetheless, the costs of these programs may or may not be above your budget. Here is where designing your own plans based on their weight-loss plans comes handy. Whether you're a beginner or professional in developing weight-loss plans, it's not as hard as it sounds.

A very compelling fact about designing your weight-loss plans is you have the luxury of creating it, just as you desire. Nonetheless, this doesn't mean you add anything and everything you wish. Especially the diet that may not even benefit you in the long run. Most of us want to lose weight for the short term benefits. However, you must always primarily consider the long-term benefits.

While losing weight can make you feel better about yourself, it can also keep you healthy in the long run. Thus, choosing a healthy way of losing weight. Here is where designing a healthy weight-loss plan comes handy. Lucky for you, the internet is your best friend.

Developing your plan requires you to do intense research, along with considering a multitude of components. Remember that not every weight-loss plan may work well for you. The very basis of a weight-loss plan is eating healthy food.

Nonetheless, most people struggle with this factor. Why, you ask?

Well, most individuals are unsure of what exactly they should eat. Furthermore, the thought of cooking complex meals can leave you feeling infuriated.

You can browse through an array of online sites to find healthy foods. I recommended you start by researching what types of food you should include in your diet. Starting from proteins, carbs, and healthy fats, jot down all the foods that you plan to add in your diet.

That being said, exercise is also an integral part of weight-loss. Just like diet, exercise is also something that depends on person to person. Some individuals may be able to lose weight fast by walking. On the other hand, some of you may need to do intense workouts to achieve your ideal goal.

Thus, take some time out to analyze which type of workout suits you the best. Then, make sure that you find a reliable website to get a hold on effective workouts. Even after finding a website, ensure that you have options so that you can rely on other fitness programs.

Another extremely brilliant way of finding workout programs is through YouTube videos. Several fitness enthusiasts put up high-intensity workouts on their YouTube channels.

Furthermore, you can also buy different exercise equipment via online websites. Utilizing these equipment means you can go through the product reviews to know if they are really efficient. Product reviews are unquestionably the game-changers to help you choose cost-effective and reliable products.

Once you have established which workout works the best for you, it's time to get into grinding. Plan a schedule - right from strategizing your meal plans to even choosing the type of workout for that respective day! Get smart, challenge yourself to maintain this fitness plan for a specific duration.

A handy tip is to create a well-effective outline of your workout and meal plan for every week. Weekly plans can help you easily distinguish your fitness goals. Furthermore, the likelihood of you maintaining your weekly plans is more compared to monthly plans.

That being said, you now know how the internet can be your greatest friend. You can use the internet, and it's offerings to your benefit to design a top-notch plan. Your suffering may, moreover, not end once you have established a plan. Most often, most of us are unable to follow and stick to our fitness plans.

Thus, one of the best ways of maintaining your fitness plans is- to never give up. However hard it may get, stick to your goals. Even if you are unable to sustain in the high-intensity workouts, make sure that you do at least a bit every day. At the end of the day, consistency is the key to losing weight.

CHAPTER 8

Is A Colon Cleanse Beneficial For Weight-Loss?

If you're a fitness freak, you might already be aware of weight loss pills. Diet pills are quite famous when it comes to losing weight. However, choosing the right diet pills for your weight-loss journey is an essential criterion for losing weight. Here, we are going to discover more about weight loss cleanses, also known as colon cleanses.

Colon cleanses, in brief, are a unique weight-loss procedure. Most individuals are still wondering if these cleanses really work. You need to note that there is a wide range of colon cleansing variants. Thus, some of these may work for you, while some of them may not.

You might come across most of these colon cleanses through advertisements. Going through the instructions beforehand while using colon cleanses is very crucial. This is because many colons cleanse are quite particular about maintaining some instructions before utilizing them.

Many colon cleanse require you to avoid eating for over one to two days. These are most often liquid formatted colon cleanses. When utilizing these, you have to ensure eating only certain types of foods.

If you are not open to buying a colon cleanse that restricts you to a particular diet, avoid it. However, If you want to ensure that the colon cleanse works magnificently, following the instructions is vital. The sole diet limitation is what makes these colon cleanses twice more effective.

A colon cleanse plays an imperative role in detoxifying your body. Thus, the colon cleanses work to mitigate different toxins from your intestine and colon. While this is an unhealthy way of losing weight, it does help in losing weight.

Every average individual has about four to eight pounds of toxins and waste stored in the body. A colon cleanses effectively helps in cleansing your body and eliminating this waste. Due to this, the colon cleanses are well-recognized as a weight-loss promoting element.

Colon cleanses that work in about three to seven days can help you encounter a swift weight-loss process. You may have already used these cleanses to lose weight before a special event happening in your life. While it is obvious that you may encounter a significant loss of weight, you should proceed with caution.

However, you will instantly get back to your earlier shape if you stop following the eating instructions. Usually, when you are asked to limit your meal plans during the colon cleanse, you may tend to shift back. While you can go back to your old eating habits, you must cut down or even eliminate your junk intake.

That being said, it comes as no surprise that losing weight through colon cleanse is very well possible. Thus, you can unquestionably give it a try. However, you must ensure that you buy only the most quality colon cleanses.

Every interested individual should go through the product reviews before buying their ideal colon cleanses. Further, also go through the instructions to analyze if you will be able to follow them.

CHAPTER 9

Are Weight Loss Pills As Effective As They Claim To Be?

Most of us have thought about utilizing weight loss pills into our diet at least once. The thing about them is that they can sound appealing to someone who will do anything to lose weight. Today, we will analyze and discover if weight loss pills are really as reliable as they claim to be.

Analyzing if weight-loss pills might benefit you requires you to consider a myriad of elements. Luckily, the factors mentioned in this book can help you get a clear understanding of weight loss pills.

The very first factor of adding weight loss pills to your fitness plan is to analyze if you are working out enough. Consuming only weight loss pills to lose weight is a myth we all want to believe in. However, weight-loss pills truly work when you blend them with other weight-loss strategies.

Most people are fast to believe that working out can be tedious and difficult. However, that's not the case. You can make your workouts twice more fun-loving if you really work into it. Moreover, if you're genuinely not enjoying your workout, chances are you may not have found your ideal workout plan.

Another very daunting factor has got to be your meal plan. How do your eating habits look like? This is a question you should undeniably ask yourself before utilizing diet pills. Adding veggies and essential proteins into your diet is a must if you want a healthy weight loss journey.

You must ensure considering these factors before trying diet pills. Naturally, losing weight for a significant amount of time is a must before trying additional methods like diet pills.

Most people tend to gain the weight back after losing it. Well, one of the chief factors for this is their eating habits. Thus, understanding why you may tend to overeat or where exactly you're going wrong is crucial.

You might have already heard the saying, 'your body fools you into thinking you're hungry most often.' I might sound ridiculous right now, but most often, we tend to overeat out of boredom. Thus, here is where weight loss pills come handy.

Many weight loss pills are known to suppress your hunger. Not only are they beneficial for suppressing your hunger, but they can also help you cut down your calorie intake. Furthermore, they also help in detecting if your body is really hungry or you're simply bored.

There are countless reasons why you might be eating out of boredom. Thus, if you want to mitigate this factor, appetite suppressants may benefit you.

Another crucial factor you need to consider is whether you are ready for the side effects of the diet pills.

The thing about diet pills is that they all vary from one another. Different Diet pills comprise varied ingredients. Due to this, every diet pill may come with different side effects.

Some of the most well-known side effects of diet pills include- dizziness, nausea, headache, irritability, jitters, anxiety, and muscle tension. Some other side effects include- insomnia, constipation, and dry mouth. This usually happens due to the chemicals that interact with your sleeping patterns.

Furthermore, suppressants are also known to prompt your nervous system. This can, in turn, enhance the heart rate and blood pressure of your body. Furthermore, it can lead to cardiac arrest or a heart attack.

People suffering from irregular heartbeat, heart diseases, and high blood pressure must consult their doctor before using diet pills. Pills like orlistat are well-known for eliminating fats through the intestines. These can cause gas, uncomfortable cramping, and even diarrhea.

If you don't already know, diet pills can substantially reduce your body's nutrient and vitamin intake. Thus, individuals interested in taking these pills should also add multivitamin supplements to their diet.

Coming to the Herbal diet pills, they are known as all-natural pills. Nonetheless, they can come with some hazardous side effects. Thus, don't mislead yourself into believing that herbal means safe.

Summing everything up, diet pills might feel like an ideal solution to weight loss. Nonetheless, they can drastically lower your caloric intake, thereby slowing down your metabolism. Thus, this leads to slowing down your weight loss rate.

Thus, considering weight loss pills for the long-term may not be ideal. You should instead look into gradually altering your lifestyle changes. Some of these include- healthy eating, consistently working out, and even marinating a proper sleep schedule.

Lastly, note that you must take some time out to do meticulous research while buying diet pills. Diet pills often come with side effects and other inconveniences. Make sure that you get an idea of how secure the pills you choose to buy are.

CHAPTER 10

Developing An Efficient Weekly Workout Program

As previously stated, a weekly program is much more adaptable when it comes to losing weight. It can help you in consistently working towards accomplishing your fitness goals.

While you may successfully plan your weekly workout program, sticking to it can be quite daunting. Thus, you must include a strategy while planning your workout program. This program should be the basis of your motivation and consistency. That being said, you must consult your doctor about your designed workout plan beforehand.

An essential and deciding component for your ideal exercise plan is to add consistent breaks for stretching. Why should you stretch? Well, to avoid soreness or potential injuries, stretching before and after your workout is essential.

Furthermore, most people tend to start their weight-loss journey by adding tedious workouts. Note that you should always start slow. Make sure to add long walks in the initial days of your workout.

The next few days, slowly increase your workout pace. For instance, you can focus your second day only on your upper body. On the third day, focus on your lower body.

Moreover, give yourself some rest on the fourth or fifth day. Start your next day with low-intensity workouts. Then, increase your pace again. Like I said, your workout should revolve around low and high-intensity exercises.

Another effective tip is to add a variety to your workout. Don't just depend on one single type of exercise. Instead, explore your options. You can swim one day, cycle the next, and so on.

This was a mere example of how you can make your workout plan a bit more exciting and less exhausting. You can alter this fitness plan based on your schedule. However, try maintaining a healthy fitness program to encounter speedy results.

CHAPTER 11

A Glimpse Into Weight Loss Supplements

Weight loss supplements are majorly used by most fitness enthusiasts. An apparent report suggests that people spend thousands of dollars regularly for buying supplements. While the fitness instructor is encountering augmented growth, finding quality supplements is still a struggle.

In the United States of America, over 30% of individuals are considered obese, and 50% overweight. While over 50 million people in the USA are trying to lose weight, only 5% are actually successful.

So, why exactly is losing weight so difficult for most of us? In all honesty, it's because we haven't found the right weight-loss hacks yet. While dietary supplements can come handy, people are quick to jump from one to another for solely encountering quick results.

A few of the common weight loss supplements that you might come across include-

- Hydrocut
- Guar Gum
- Diet Patch
- Magnetic Diet Pills
- Electrical Muscle stimulators
- Weight loss earrings (no, Just joking)
- Garcinia Cambogia Extract
- Orlistat (Alli)
- While all of these supplements claim to offer effective results, they aren't worth buying. You will also come across numerous diet drinks. However, these are only effective for short-term weight-loss goals.

A few of the diet drinks that you might come across include

- Ultra Slim Fast
- Shakeology
- Black Tea
- Apple Cider Vinegar Drinks
- Ginger Tea
- High-Protein Drink
- Nestle's Sweet Success
- Wonder slim
- Super Lean Shots

Herbalife Nutritional Program

Next are the herbal remedies. While these remedies claim to offer safe weight loss results, they only offer short-term benefits. Let's discover a few of them in-depth.

·   Chromium Supplements- Claim to reduce blood sugar levels, cholesterol, and fat. However, they can cause anemia most often.

·   Algae Tablets- These tablets comprise a prominent amount of nutrients. These offer effective results but are quite heftily priced.

·   Green Tea Extracted products- They are well-known for their robust antioxidant properties for lowering triglycerides and cholesterol. They are further known for driving weight loss. However, the caffeine content may adversely affect the users and further cause restlessness and insomnia.

·   Glucomannan products- Suggests that consume two pills before every meal can help you lower your food absorption. It is further known as a food thickener. However, it isn't scientifically proven to be efficient or safe and may only offer results on maintaining a strict diet.

- St John's Wort Supplement- It claims to suppress your food absorption. However, it comes with several side effects. Some of these include- sleeplessness, discomfort, tiredness, and gastrointestinal issues.

Some manufactures also claim that their products comprise of EGCG. EGCG is a distinctive ingredient extracted from Green Tea. The component is known for speeding up the weight loss process.

The exact effects of ECGC are still unknown. I would summarize that Green Tea doesn't account for a solitary weight-loss solution. However, you can add it to your diet plan for reducing tissue fat.

Furthermore, it also enhances thermo-Genesis and day oxidation. It then acts as a fast fat-burning element and promotes your metabolism rate.

Experts are trying to discover several other noteworthy perks of EGCG. Some of them include benefits for cholesterol, blood sugar, bad breath, and much more.

To summarize this, you must consult your doctor before using supplements. Furthermore, make sure to thoroughly go through the details and benefits of every supplement before you buy it.

CHAPTER 12

Can Hypnosis Significantly Work As A Weight-Loss Treatment?

One of the most common factors that most of us struggle with is maintaining our weight. Preventing yourself from gaining excess weight is an integral factor in avoiding future health issues.

If you aren't already aware, weight over 20 pounds than your required weight can put you at an increased health risk. Some of these health risks include- obstructive sleep apnea, coronary heart disease, and even breast cancer.

If you live a very inactive lifestyle, your likelihood of gaining excess weight is more. Moreover, if you are inactive and overweight, you may expose yourself to hazardous risks like cardiovascular disease. On the other hand, losing weight can mitigate such risks.

On the bright side, losing even a minimal amount of weight can significantly benefit you. Thanks to the evolution of technology, you will come across vast methods of weight loss. One such procedure that you may be familiar with is hypnosis.

Nonetheless, several controversial misconceptions are being discussed subject to hypnosis. Since hypnosis doesn't revolve around any type of drug or medication, most people prefer it for weight loss.

If you choose to go ahead with hypnosis for weight loss, you should consider getting to know more about the treatment. We will discover some of the fundamental insights of hypnosis.

Hypnosis can be extremely hazardous if done by an unprofessional individual. While several people think hypnosis may not adversely affect your health, you may need to reconsider. Choosing a high-trained and skilled individual for your hypnosis treatment is necessary.

That being said, merely utilizing hypnosis for weight loss is not sufficient. Many experts suggest that this treatment shouldn't be the only method utilized for weight loss.

Furthermore, not that a single hypnosis session may not be sufficient for your ideal results. Experts suggest that psychotherapy and hypnosis together can help you achieve milestones of results.

Hypnosis is the deliberate procedure of accessing the subliminal state of an individual. The body of an individual is comparatively more responsive when in a subliminal stage.

Needless to say, hypnosis cannot entirely reprogram your mind to eliminate your junk intake. In a nutshell, hypnosis is quite a natural and soothing state of your mind that only occurs twice a day. We may chiefly experience this euphoric state right before falling asleep or even before fully waking up.

When you choose hypnosis as an alternative weight loss treatment, it brainwashes your mind into healthy eating. These suggestions further fortify to replace your bad habits with good ones.

Several individuals suggest that hypnosis worked well for them to establish a healthy lifestyle. Hypnosis is an excellent way of offering sharp subconscious suggestions.

At the end of the day, a healthy mind means a healthy body. You should, however, consult your doctor for the right eating and exercising suggestions.

CHAPTER 13

Joining A Paid Weight Loss Program

Thanks to the abundant weight loss programs, you have the choice of choosing from a vast availability. The most popular means of weight loss plans include designing your own plan and paying for one.

If you're just starting your weight loss journey, you should instead work on making your own plan. You can play with different plans to analyze which of them may benefit you maximally. To do so, start by determining the pros and cons of different weight loss plans that you choose to consider.

Several online platforms, such as Weight Watchers and Nutrisystem, offer versatile weight loss plans. While these may be paid plans, they can benefit you tremendously.

Joining a weight loss program means attending different meetings, discussions, and whatnot. While it might sound exhausting, you will have a real chance of losing weight. Furthermore, you can also get your hands on healthy meal plans.

The best part about weight loss programs is that you will have hands-on professional programs. Thus, your chance of losing weight can drastically increase. Furthermore, these programs are entirely based on your convenience.

In most cases, individual trainers help every individual through their weight loss journey. With well-equipped professionals by your side, losing weight can become effortlessly easy.

Thus, the only setback of paying for weight loss programs is the money you need to pay. Thus, choosing a weight loss program is entirely on you. Are you willing to pay a certain amount for losing weight? Or do you think you can lose weight on your own?

Nonetheless, nobody should have to put themselves under a financial strain for losing weight via paid workout programs. There is a plethora of ways to lose weight, as we previously discussed.

Another appealing feature of a paid workout program is that you can personalize them. For instance, you can choose the meal plans based on your likeliness of the food.

On the bright side, designing your own workouts can also extensively benefit you. You can do thorough research to ensure choosing only the most suitable meal plans and workouts. You can then incorporate them into your weight loss journey.

Furthermore, designing your own meal plan gives you the convenience and flexibility of time. Unlike weight loss programs, you can choose to work out or even eat whenever you're potentially free.

Moreover, you can also check out different websites online to plan your weight loss plan according to your convenience. In the long run, you will also fall in love with researching what your body needs to lose weight.

The bottom line is that choosing your own weight-loss plan, or a paid weight-loss plan is entirely up to you. However, make sure that you don't forget to have fun. Make your weight loss journey all about loving yourself through the process.

Lastly, whatever you choose, consistently working out, and eating healthy is the key to losing weight.

CHAPTER 14

The Dangers Associated With Rapid Weight Loss

Most of us are eager and quite fast to find rapid weight loss techniques. Rapid weight loss or quick weight loss is the process of losing weight at a comparatively faster pace. In brief, this can range from anything between two to seven days.

Every year, thousands of people are attracted to fast weight loss techniques. From wanting to lose weight before an event to much more, losing weight speedily is something we all wish for.

While you can find several ways to lose weight in no time, you need to be extremely cautious. Moreover, rapid weight loss is a very unhealthy approach to weight loss. In the long run, you will undeniably gain back the weight loss through speedy weight loss techniques.

Most of us are guilty of starving ourselves to lose weight. Starving yourself or eating less than your body requires can drastically impact your health. You could instead focus on eating healthy and eliminate junk food from your eating habits.

Sometimes, we even tend to eat less for the amount of exercise we do. For instance, you may work out for over 3 hours a day and eat fewer calories. Such attempts for losing weight will backfire you in the near future.

Another explicitly infuriating component related to rapid weight loss is the intake of different weight-loss supplements. While you will come across several safe and effective supplements, you cannot entirely depend on them.

Thus, if you really want to go ahead with weight loss supplements, you should do extensive research before buying them. This research can revolve around anything from reading product reviews and consulting a healthcare specialist.

With that being said, note that seeking help from professionals is extremely important for a healthy weight loss journey. You cannot blindly give into different supplements and meal plans before knowing anything about them. While you cannot hide from the upcoming essential events, do not choose unhealthy weight-loss techniques.

If you really want to go ahead with rapid weight loss, no one can stop you. However, you should also note that there are numerous risks linked to it.

The bottom line is that losing weight is undeniably full of challenges. You will give up several times before you learn to stay consistent. However, I know that losing weight is not impossible.

In fact, if you truly dedicate yourself to work hard, you will notice results in no time. However, working hard is not as easy as it sounds. You will have to give up on your unhealthy habits. From sleeping on time, eating healthy, and even working out.

How you choose to lose weight is entirely up to you. No one can judge you for it. However, lose weight fundamentally for becoming fit and healthy. It is essential that you consider long-term goals and not just the short-term ones.

If you want to enhance your quality of life and if you think losing weight can help you boost your self-esteem, it can. At the end of the day, it is all based on your perspective and mindset.

CONCLUSION

Follow this book if you're willing to lose weight for you and you only. I just want to say that everybody should love their bodies the way they are. You need to feel comfortable in your skin too, and if you're not, then you could try different ways to change that.

This book is only for the people who need help reducing weight as the extra weight can be dangerous to their health. This journey is not going to be easy, but remember- it gets worse before it can get better. Be kinder to yourself and forgive yourself for not meeting your expectations.

Take this journey one at a time and be your biggest cheerleader. Motivate yourself to do better, and in no time, you will see the changes you desired.

ADDITIONAL RESOURCES

Hot Skinny Tea - Detox Tea For Weight Loss!

https://bit.ly/2ZEfWh

Always Eat After 7PM Book

https://bit.ly/32vyYIC

Living Healthy With Chocolate

https://bit.ly/2WAp0C1

PROVEN-weight loss and body detoxifying supplements

https://bit.ly/2DQMkoA

Do you have stored body fat that you have tried to get rid of in the past, but nothing worked?

https://bit.ly/3jiAfJ5